Beyond Trauma

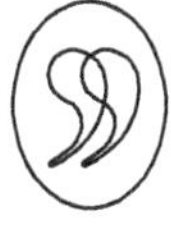

Beyond Trauma

CHRISTEL PRATER

StoryTerrace

Design StoryTerrace

First print August 2024

StoryTerrace

www.StoryTerrace.com

CONTENTS

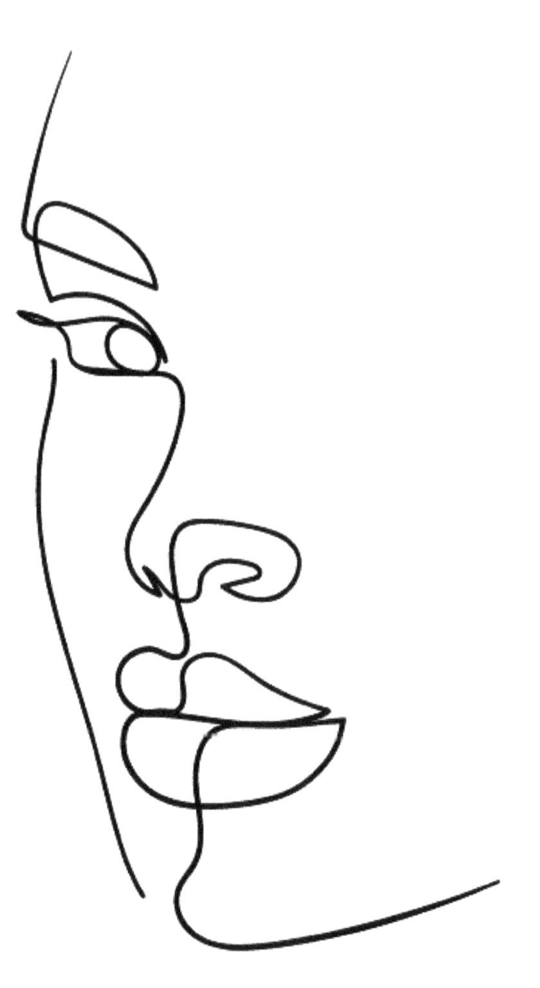

1

INTRODUCTION

The room fell silent as I spoke. Tears were streaming down my face, my heart pounding in my chest. I had never shared the truth about my marriage before; it had been hard enough admitting it to myself. But here I was, at a Bible retreat, finally sharing the painful reality I had been living with for so long.

My voice shaking, I revealed the emotional abuse I had been living with for years. Our marriage became so toxic that I didn't know how much longer I could take it.

As I shared more details of the trauma I had endured, I glanced over at my husband, expecting to see some flicker of emotion, some acknowledgment of the pain he had caused. But his face remained stone cold. There was not a tear in his eyes, not a hint of remorse in his expression.

Everything changed with that one glance. At that moment, something shifted inside me. I realized I couldn't continue living like this, couldn't keep sacrificing my own well-being for a marriage that was slowly destroying me—

emotionally, mentally, and physically. I wanted out.

But leaving a toxic marriage is never easy, especially when you're a Christian woman. For years, several people in my church had been telling me I needed to stay; that divorce was not an option.

"Draw a line in the sand and move forward," they said. "Let it go."

Their words weighed heavy on my heart. I knew they meant well, but they didn't understand the depths of the trauma I was experiencing. They couldn't see the emotional scars that were hidden beneath the surface. I wouldn't let them. Until that Bible retreat, I hadn't told anyone.

As I struggled with the decision to leave, I found myself drawn to the Bible story in John chapter 4 of the woman at the well. Here was a woman who had five husbands, and was living with a man who wasn't her husband. By all accounts, she was an outcast, someone to be shunned and judged.

But when Jesus met her at the well, he didn't condemn her. He didn't tell her to go back to her husband, to stick it out no matter how difficult things got. Instead, he offered her living water, a chance to start anew.

"Go and sin no more," he told her. And with those words, he set her free.

That story spoke volumes to me as I went through my own divorce. I realized that so many women in the church stay in toxic marriages because they're afraid of being criticized, of being seen as a failure. They've been told by pastors or fellow church members that leaving is unbiblical and that they need to submit to their husbands no matter what.

But that's not what Jesus modeled for us. He came to set the captives free, to bind up the brokenhearted. And sometimes, that means walking away from a situation that is causing us harm.

As I navigated the painful process of divorce, I clung to my faith like a lifeline. I prayed for strength, for guidance, for healing. And slowly but surely, I began to emerge from the darkness.

It wasn't an easy journey. There were days when I wondered if I would ever feel whole again, if I would ever be able to trust another person with my heart. But through therapy, through leaning into my relationship with God, I began to heal.

Now, I can look back on that time in my life with a sense of gratitude. Not for the trauma itself, but for the growth that came from it. I am a different person now—stronger, wiser, more compassionate. And I have a burning desire to help others who are walking through similar struggles.

That's why I decided to write this book. As a certified mental health coach and life coach with two communication degrees, I have the training and experience to guide others on their own healing journeys. But more than that, I have the personal experience of living through trauma and coming out the other side.

In these pages, I will share my own stories of pain and

resilience. But this book is not just about me. It's about you, too. At the end of each chapter, you'll find coaching questions and exercises designed to help you process your own experiences and take steps toward healing.

We'll delve into the importance of mindset, exploring how our thoughts and beliefs shape our reality. We'll talk about setting boundaries, about learning to love ourselves, about forgiving those who have hurt us. We'll grapple with tough questions like whether to stay in a difficult situation or leave and how to rebuild our lives on whichever path we take.

My goal is that by the end of this book, you'll have a framework for moving forward, no matter what your specific circumstances may be. Whether you choose to stay in your current situation or make a fresh start, you'll have the tools you need to reclaim your story and create a life that feels authentic and fulfilling.

As I sit here writing these words, I am reminded of a quote that has become a mantra for me in recent years: "If you don't like your life, you can change it. You are the author of your own story."

For so long, I felt like my story was being written by other people—by my now ex-husband, by well-meaning but misguided church leaders, by societal expectations of what a "good Christian wife" should be. But now I know the truth: I am the only one, with God's guidance, who gets to decide how my story unfolds.

And the same is true for you. No matter what hardships

you have faced, no matter how many times you have felt powerless or uncertain in your direction, you always have the power to choose what comes next. You can pick up the pen that others have tried to wrestle from your hands and start writing a new chapter.

It won't be easy. Healing from trauma is hard, messy, non-linear work. There will be setbacks and discouragements along the way. But I promise you this: It is so worth it. Because on the other side of that journey is a life that is richer, more authentic, and more joyful than you ever could have imagined.

So take a deep breath, dear reader. Turn the page. And let's begin this brave, beautiful work together.

In the next chapter, we'll take a closer look at what it means to live in trauma—the signs to watch for, the different ways it can manifest, and the devastating toll it can take on our minds, bodies, and spirits. This may be painful territory to explore, but it is a crucial first step on the road to healing. Stay with me, friend. Freedom is coming.

Chapter 1 Homework

Go to God in prayer before you begin answering the following questions. Ask him to prepare you for this time and to share his wisdom and desires for your life.

1. Reflect: What do you hope to accomplish as you journey through this book?
2. Assess: Describe your current situation and what problems you are facing.
3. Affirm: Write a personal promise to yourself outlining the goals you want to achieve through this book.
4. Connect: Take a moment to pray and silently seek God's guidance and wisdom for your circumstance.
5. Commit: Prioritize making a change in your life by scheduling dedicated time to engage with this workbook. Be specific.

Days of the week: ______________

Time: ______________

Place: ______________

Additional Insights

Every relationship has its ups and downs. It's important to understand this cycle of positive and negative, good and bad, and recognize that neither phase lasts forever.

As parents, we make sacrifices to shield our children and close family members from the bad times. As a result, they rarely see the big picture and tend to only remember the good times.

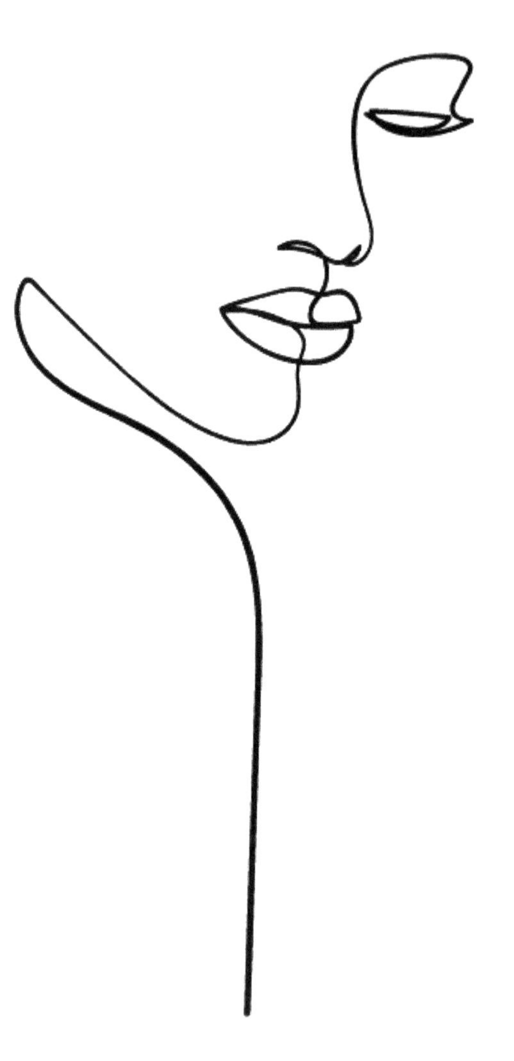

2

LIVING IN TRAUMA

Growing up, I didn't know any different. My parents, while I believe they loved me deep down, didn't know how to properly express that love. They were abusive and neglectful, leaving me with deep wounds and feelings of low self-esteem and self-worth that would persist well into adulthood. One time when I was only seven years old, my mom slapped me out of a chair because I was having trouble tying my shoe. Another time as a teenager, my dad kicked me down a flight of stairs. Those memories, that trauma, sticks with you.

Desperate for security, comfort, and what I thought was love, I married young to an older man. I was only 19 and he was eight years my senior. People warned me at the time to stay away from him, that his temper was dangerous. But I was pregnant and felt obligated to make it work for my child. When that didn't magically fix things between us, I got pregnant again, still hoping it would bring us closer. It didn't.

What followed was nine years of physical, verbal, and emotional trauma that grew more volatile over time. I can still picture the exact chair I was sitting in the day he flew into a rage and threw a coffee table clear across our living room at me. I'll never forget where I was standing, shaking, the day he pulled a gun on me—the final straw that made me grab my kids and flee.

In the tumultuous divorce that followed, he actually took my children. He told them I was in jail as an excuse for why they couldn't see me. It took me six agonizing months to get them back. Through it all, even though I had fallen away from regularly attending church, I leaned heavily on my faith to get me through. My pastor at the time, Pastor Doug, helped me see that I had biblical grounds to divorce my husband. He showed me the scriptures that spoke about God not condoning violence and His desire for my protection and peace. It was the validation and clarity I needed to move forward.

While I worked two jobs to support us, my ex-husband and his family came one day and cleaned out our entire house, loading everything into U-Hauls while I was gone. They even took my work clothes, leaving only the unpaid furniture behind. I came home to an empty house and had to call the police in tears. They said I couldn't even stay there that night because it was considered a crime scene. With no family in the area, I had to ask a friend if I could sleep on her couch. It was a low and traumatic point.

After licking my wounds from that marriage, I was single for about six years before meeting husband number two. This time would be different, I told myself, because I met him at church, at a small-group event. We started dating and while there were red flags, like him making an offhand comment early on that I "almost fit his cookie cutter" of what he was looking for and frequently putting his son and ex-wife's needs and wants above mine, I ignored them. I thought meeting him in the safety of the church meant God had orchestrated this relationship and it would be the godly, healthy marriage I longed for.

I was wrong. Within our first year of marriage, we were already in counseling. He actually walked out on one of our sessions, despite the counselor telling him he had issues he needed to work on. The counselor even said to me that since I didn't have kids with this man yet, I should seriously consider leaving. But I stuffed down that gnawing in my gut. I wanted so desperately to be the good Christian wife who could make her marriage work. I kept hoping and praying he would change, that I could change him.

But his toxic, narcissistic behaviors only escalated. There was betrayal, like the time he agreed to let a repair person into our rental house after I had expressly said no because I had a sick child at home. He was on the phone with her, looked right at me, and turned his back to me to tell her that yes, she could come. He completely disregarded my wishes and authority as his wife. The broken promises were endless—he would say sorry but never change. Rinse and repeat in a crazy-making cycle.

I fell into a destructive pattern with him, of him waking me up in the middle of the night, not for any emergency, but simply because he wanted to pick a fight. It would start with him saying something like, "I don't want to argue but . . ." and then purposely pushing my buttons until we were in a heated argument that would end with him guilting me into having sex with him, always on his terms with no regard for my wants or needs. The whole manipulative, toxic cycle would repeat every few weeks. I later learned this is a common narcissistic abuse tactic.

Through my training as a mental health coach, I learned about the cycle of trauma and how abuse often follows a specific pattern of tension building, an explosive incident, a honeymoon period, and then a calm before it starts all over again. I lived this cycle on repeat for years:

Key elements are: Tension Building -> Incident -> Reconciliation (Honeymoon Period) -> Calm -> Tension Building, in a circle.

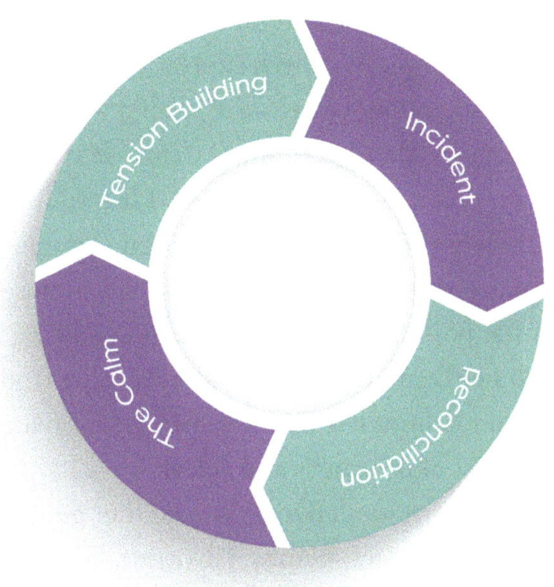

Living in this continual trauma warps your mind and erodes your sense of self. You have to actively change the way you think—about yourself, your abuser, your expectations—in order to break free. For so long, I tricked myself into believing I deserved this treatment, that I was the problem, and that if I just tried harder or was a better wife, he would finally treat me with love and respect. I allowed everyone to chip away at my self-worth until I hardly recognized myself. You have to raise the value you place on yourself or you'll be doomed to continue in the cycle of abuse.

So why did I stay so long, enabling my own trauma? At first, I made excuses, telling myself I had to keep trying to make it work for the kids' sake. I was worried about being judged by friends, family, and my church if I divorced again. I had so many people at church simply telling me to "draw a line in the sand and move forward," as if it were that simple. They couldn't see that I was slowly dying on the inside.

Finances were a huge worry as well. I feared how I would support myself and my children if I left. Despite being a successful career woman, my self-worth had been so ground down by that point that I couldn't imagine making it on my own. I also held onto the misguided belief that God wanted me to remain committed to my marriage no matter what, even at the cost of my sanity and safety.

At my core, I just wanted to be seen as the "good Christian wife" with the perfect family. Divorced, abused women didn't fit that mold, so I climbed into it and tried to quietly disappear. I ignored all the warnings and red flags, brushing off concerned friends and family, convinced I could single-handedly change him if I just loved harder, submitted more, and kept showing up like a good churchgoing wife and mother.

What I couldn't admit at the time was how little I valued myself. I had no self-worth left. Through the toxic cycles of abuse, the most important lesson I had to learn was to value myself again as a woman made in the image of God. My faith had to shift from an allegiance to the institution of marriage to a trust in a God who loved me too much to see me destroyed by abuse. I had to raise my expectations of how I deserved to be treated and learn to love myself. Until I did that critical heart and head work, I would remain firmly stuck in trauma. With each cycle, we continue to grow more destructive.

God doesn't want us living in trauma. He tells us this through the Bible story of the woman caught in adultery whom the Pharisees drag before Jesus. Society condemned her and wanted her punished. We can still get caught up in the fear of condemnation today. We're conditioned to believe that if we don't go along with what people are telling us to do, then we'll be cast aside.

But Jesus, the only one who had the right to condemn this woman, did the opposite, and instead turned to her accusers and famously said, "Let any one of you who is without sin cast the first stone." After they all eventually skulked away, He looked at her with pure love and declared, "Then neither do I condemn you. Now go and sin no more." He didn't send her back to her old way of life because he knew she had a better future ahead of her. He acknowledged her inherent dignity, affirmed her value, and freed her from shame to step into a brand-new life. This is the same gracious healing and restoration Jesus longs to give each of us.

As Jeremiah 29:11 reminds us "'For I know the plans I have for you,' declares the Lord, 'plans to prosper you and not to harm you, plans to give you hope and a future.'" Regardless of your age or stage of life, it is never too late to start writing a courageous new chapter. Pace yourself and hold your judgments about yourself loosely. Wherever you sense God's delight and the desires He's placed within you, have the audacity to dream bigger than your past.

My journey of choosing to live free from abuse was not a single choice, but a series of small, holy yeses—to myself, my children, my future, and my God. With each brave boundary and hard decision, I took back more control over my own life and began to see myself as a woman worthy of love and respect.

The cycle of abuse can feel impossible to break free from, but I am living proof that change is possible when you begin to see your own beautiful value again. In the next chapter, I'll share more about the choices that led to my freedom and healing. Because as long as you have breath in your lungs, you have choices.

Chapter 2 Homework

Go to God in prayer before you begin answering the following questions. Ask him to prepare you for this time and to share his wisdom and desires for your life.

1. Reflect: Have you experienced any childhood traumas that have continued to affect you as an adult? If so, list them below.
2. Assess: Of the traumas you listed, did any of them seem normal or acceptable at the time?

3. Explore: If you stayed in a traumatic situation in the past, what was your reason for staying? If you are in a traumatic situation currently, why do you stay?
4. Analyze: Consider the cycle of trauma described in this chapter and apply it to your own life. Can you identify repeated behaviors? Do you see this cycle occurring at different stages of your life?
5. Focus: Which aspects of this chapter resonated with you the most? List them below.
6. Pray: Ask God for wisdom to help you clearly recognize the traumas and toxic situations in your life and to guide you in making healthy choices.
7. Reflect: Take time alone to contemplate the traumatic situations you are addressing. Identify the most distressing areas and imagine how your life would be without these toxic behaviors cycling through. List your reflections below.

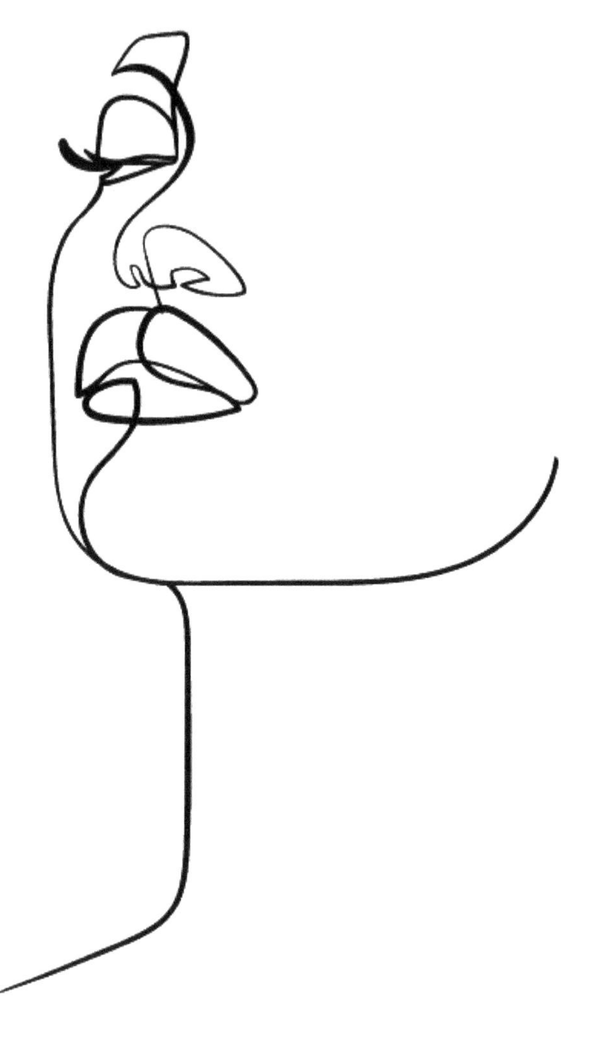

3

YOU HAVE CHOICES

Why am I choosing to stay in this trauma? That was the question swirling in my head as I sat in the group session at the five-day couples' retreat, my husband stone-faced and emotionless beside me while I unraveled, revealing for the first time the depth of pain and abuse I had endured.

The other couples in the room wept with compassion and shock. But my husband, the one who had betrayed and violated my most intimate boundaries, remained unmoved. And in that moment, something inside me broke. I could no longer ignore the truth staring me in the face—love does not behave this way. I deserved better. I deserved to be cherished and protected, not used and disrespected.

Yet even with this realization, I hesitated. I feared the unknown that came with finally walking away. Was it my faith holding me back? The subtle and not-so-subtle messages from my church that divorce was a sin, a black mark against my character?

"Draw a line in the sand and move forward," they told me when I went to them for counsel. As if it were that simple. As if I could erase years of trauma and pain with a simple flick of the wrist.

Or maybe it was the judgment I feared from family and friends. I had been down this road of divorce once before and knew all too well the whispers that would follow. The pity. The condemnation that I had "failed" yet again at the institution of marriage. Never mind that I was the one being abused. Never mind that I was the one pouring everything I had into trying to make it work, even as pieces of myself crumbled in the process.

If I'm being completely honest, my reasons for staying imprisoned in a toxic marriage for so long really boiled down to one thing—fear. Bone-deep, paralyzing fear of the unknown. Of being alone. Of trying to make it financially on my own. The insecurities that told me I wasn't good enough, that I didn't deserve better, kept me rooted in place even as my very soul withered.

So I made excuses. I became the master of putting my own needs last. When my father fell ill with terminal cancer, I convinced myself I had to be the dutiful daughter and caretaker. I couldn't possibly pursue a divorce during this time—it would be selfish. Then my daughter's and son's health deteriorated, and I poured all my energy into helping them get well. Before I knew it, years had slipped by in this fog of caretaking and people-pleasing. Years I could never get back.

All the while, the stress and trauma continued to take its toll. What started as emotional and verbal abuse escalated until even my body began to rebel under the strain. Chronic pain, autoimmune issues, and tumors that required multiple surgeries to remove. I see now that I was literally making myself sick trying to light myself on fire to keep everyone else warm. But at the time, I couldn't see the forest for the trees. I had lost myself so completely that I didn't know which way was up anymore.

Rock bottom came in the form of yet another argument with my husband. But this time, instead of cowering and apologizing, something in me snapped. Enough was enough. I was done living as a shell of myself, taking crumbs and calling it a feast. I didn't want to wake up 20 years from now, looking back on my life with regret that I let someone else control my story. It was time to reclaim my power, terrifying as that was.

But here's the thing, sweet friend. You always have a choice. No matter how trapped you may feel, or how hopeless your circumstances seem, you get to decide what comes next. Because let me tell you, living in resentment that your choices have been taken from you is just another form of victimhood. One that will rob you of true peace and joy if you let it.

When I finally made the decision to leave and pursue a divorce, I braced myself for the rejection. The harsh words and judgment that I felt certain would come. Yes, it was an adjustment and there were bumps along the way. But my family understood on a fundamental level that Mom needed to do this for her own well-being. They saw the light slowly returning to my eyes and knew it was worth any temporary hardship.

As for friends and family? I quickly learned who was truly in my corner and who was simply there for the gossip fodder. And while it hurt to let some people go, I knew I was making room for relationships built on mutual love, respect, and understanding. The fear of being alone has a funny way of tricking us into settling for far less than we deserve.

I share all of this not to cast blame or play the victim card, but rather to illustrate that mindset is everything when it comes to breaking free and creating a new life after trauma. Are you going to view this next chapter as an adventure to cherish or an obstacle to overcome? Will you choose to see the rejection as a reflection of your worth or simply a redirection to something better? These are the types of questions I had to answer as I pieced myself back together.

It starts with giving yourself permission to want more. To dare to dream of a life that sets your soul on fire, even if it looks different than what you originally planned. Forgiveness, of both yourself and those who have wronged you, is also essential. Not because they necessarily deserve it, but because you do. You deserve to lay down the heavy weight of resentment and bitterness. To step forward into the next chapter unburdened by the wounds of your past.

There comes a point where you have to decide—am I going to shrink back and settle for a half-lived life dictated by fear? Or will I allow myself to believe I am worthy of more? Of being cherished, respected, and seen? Will I continue to betray myself in order to make everyone else comfortable? These are the choices that we often don't realize we have when we're knee-deep in trauma and chaos. But I'm here to tell you that you always have options. You always get to decide what you will and won't accept moving forward.

Yes, there are consequences and uncomfortable conversations that may come with choosing to break free from a toxic situation. It's not a decision to be made flippantly. But in my experience, the price of staying silent and stuck is ultimately much higher. It robs you of hope. Of the life and love you could be experiencing. It keeps you trapped in a vicious cycle of your own making.

So I encourage you to get quiet with yourself. Look honestly at your situation and get crystal clear on what problems need addressing. Maybe it means setting firmer boundaries with your partner while you undergo counseling together. Maybe it means looking at your financial situation and getting creative about ways to support yourself if you do decide to leave. The only way out is through, as they say.

But you don't have to navigate this treacherous terrain alone. Reach out for support—whether that's a trusted counselor, a coach, or a friend who gets it. Be discerning about who you allow to speak into your situation, though.

Well-meaning as they may be, not everyone understands the nuances and complexities of relational trauma. Learning to trust my instincts and honor my own needs above all else has been a game-changer.

Ultimately, this is about so much more than just deciding whether you stay or go. It's about learning to trust yourself again. To know that you can face hard things and come out the other side stronger. It's about falling in love with the woman in the mirror and believing she is worth fighting for. Worth choosing every single day. Even when it's messy and confusing and downright terrifying.

Because that seemingly small, whispered act of declaring "I'm choosing me" is the start of everything. The moment you decide your peace, your joy, and your emotional, mental, and physical well-being come first. No more putting yourself last. No more accepting crumbs and telling yourself it's enough.

I won't lie and say that changing your mindset from victim to victor is an overnight process. There were many days I took one step forward only to slide three steps back, where I questioned everything and fought against the old, limiting beliefs that kept me stuck for so long. Healing is rarely linear. It requires a diligent commitment to showing up for yourself. To choose the empowered path again and again until it becomes second nature.

But it IS possible to get to the other side of this. To wake up one day and realize you no longer flinch at your own shadow. That you can set healthy boundaries and advocate for your needs without the choking fear of being "too much." Without worrying that the other shoe could drop at any moment. There is so much hope and beauty waiting for you in this next chapter. All you have to do is decide that you're worth it. That you're willing to do the work, have the hard conversations, and honor your own healing.

No matter where you find yourself in this journey, hear this: You have a right to take up space. To want more. To demand change if something is no longer serving you. I know it's terrifying to rock the boat, especially if you've spent your whole life trying to shove down your own needs to make others comfortable. But I promise you that when you start showing up for yourself, God has a way of rearranging to support you in ways you could never imagine. You realize you were never alone in this. Grace finds you every single time.

So what choices will you make today to honor your healing? Where are you ready to take your power back and start writing a new story? Maybe it's finally calling that counselor and setting up an appointment. Or having a heart-to-heart with your best friend about what's really been going on behind closed doors. Start there. And then do the next right thing. And the next. One baby step at a time until you've built a mountain of self-trust and a new life you can't wait to wake up to every day.

You've got this, warrior. I believe in you. More importantly, I hope you're beginning to believe in yourself, too. Because that is the single most important choice you can make—to believe you are worthy of an extraordinary life. One that doesn't require you to sacrifice your mental health or well-being. One that celebrates all of you—even the parts you once deemed "too much."

I invite you to begin exploring what your new chapter could look like. What would you create if fear was no longer a factor? If you gave yourself radical permission to want what you want without guilt or hesitation? Let yourself dream. Get carried away. There is so much magic waiting for you on the other side of deciding to choose yourself. But you have to be willing to take that first terrifying step. To say no to what is no longer serving you, so you can say hell yes to what lights you up.

You have choices. You have agency. You have the power to create a life that feels nourishing and expansive and soul-stirring, even if it looks nothing like you once imagined. Trust the tiny voice inside nudging you forward. She knows the way. All you have to do is take her hand and begin.

In the next chapter, we'll be diving into the very real and often misunderstood consequences of trauma—how it impacts our mental, emotional, and physical health in ways we may not even realize. I'll be sharing more of my own journey and the hard-won lessons I've learned along the way. Buckle up, buttercup. This is where the real work begins. But I promise you it will be so worth it. One choice at a time. One day at a time. You've got this.

Chapter 3 Homework

Go to God in prayer before you begin answering the following questions. Ask him to prepare you for this time and to share his wisdom and desires for your life.

1. Explore: What choices do you currently have in this situation?
2. Choose: Can you identify a decision you could make without outside influence? If so, what would you choose to do?
3. Examine: Which parts of your life have you put on hold in order to cope with trauma?
4. Reflect: Looking at your situation, where do you think your "rock bottom" might be, the point where you'd be willing to make difficult changes?
5. Take Inventory: Identify your top three insecurities that are hindering your ability to change.
6. Identify: If you choose to stay in your situation, what boundaries can you set to manage your top three traumas or toxic behaviors? Use the space provided at the end of this chapter to list them.
7. Clarify: If you choose to leave your current situation, what are the top three obstacles you foresee? Use the color chart provided to brainstorm potential solutions.

Traumas	Boundaries
	1. 2. 3.
	1. 2. 3.
	1. 2. 3.

8. Name: List three places or people you can turn to for support and guidance during this process.
9. Imagine: What would you want to do or be if your current situation wasn't a factor?
10. Dream: What's your favorite dream? Consider your options and the opportunities available to you and make a plan to achieve them.
11. Evaluate: Identify areas in your life where you struggle to trust yourself. List them below.
12. Define: What do you want to achieve in your current situation? Brainstorm actionable steps you can take to move closer to your desired life.
13. Pray: Spend time in prayer, using the insights gained from this chapter to guide your thoughts and decisions.

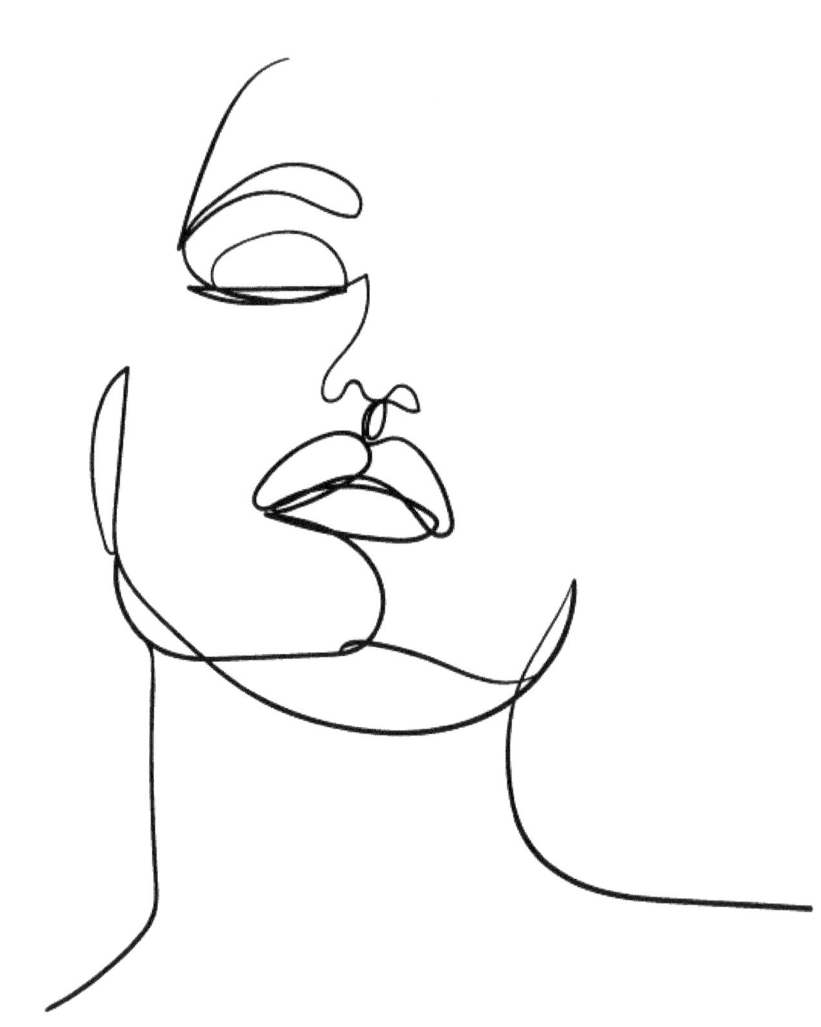

4

CONSEQUENCES OF TRAUMA

Looking back now, I see how prolonged trauma took a devastating toll on my life—physically, mentally, and emotionally. For years, I hid the signs of abuse from those closest to me out of shame. I didn't want anyone to know the reality of what I was going through behind closed doors.

But you can only mask the pain for so long before it catches up with you. The stress of living in constant trauma mode wreaked havoc on my health in all aspects. Physically, I gained a massive amount of weight, ballooning up to almost 300 pounds in my 30s and 40s during my second marriage—a time that was supposed to be the prime of my life. Instead, I was the most unhealthy and miserable I'd ever been.

My body broke down under the pressure. In a 10-year span, I underwent 20 surgeries, most of them to remove tumors and address other concerning health issues that had cropped up, likely as a result of suppressing all the trauma. I developed high blood pressure and was borderline diabetic. Stress caused silver dollar-sized bald spots in my hair. Multiple vital organs were impacted—I lost my thyroid, ovaries, and gallbladder because they had been "eaten up" by the constant cortisol and stress hormones flooding my system from holding everything inside.

Mentally and emotionally, I became disconnected from my true self and who I was. I sank into a deep depression but tried to put on a happy face for the world. Severe anxiety led to being prescribed three different heavy-duty medications—Ativan, Xanax, and Valium—all at the same time just to cope and function.

I spent years where I would cry daily but camouflage it behind a smile and laughter so no one would know the depths of my pain. My uncle used to say I could laugh among my tears, that I had a special ability to be breaking apart crying on the inside while smiling on the outside and no one could tell. It was a survival skill I had perfected.

Being immersed in the toxicity of trauma for so long caused me to normalize my husbands' narcissistic and damaging behaviors. I made excuses for their actions and took responsibility for their poor choices. Even worse, I started to pick up some of those same toxic traits and treated others poorly at times, operating out of my unhealed wounds. I became defensive, withdrawn, and would isolate myself. I didn't like who I was becoming but felt powerless to change.

Red flags and warning signs kept popping up in my marriages, but I ignored them. There were moments of clarity where I'd start to see the writing on the wall, like when I asked for a divorce in 2013 after the abuse, but then I would doubt myself and shrink back into victim mode. I didn't see a way out of the madness.

My sleep was impacted greatly by the trauma as well. I developed insomnia and would regularly wake up with panic attacks. Even now that I've been out of my marriage for some time, I still struggle some nights, waking up panicked because my brain has been rewired from all those years of trauma interrupting my rest. It shows how those wounds linger and take time to heal even after removing yourself from the situation.

The consequences of trauma run deep and will continue to negatively impact all facets of your life the longer you stay in it. I wish I had realized it sooner—that the exhaustion, depression, anger, insecurity, and health issues were all tied to the toxic relationships and environments I kept subjecting myself to. But I couldn't see clearly while in the thick of it.

You can't fix the effects of trauma on your own. I couldn't, even though I had gone through mental health coaching courses and was helping others in crisis. It was beyond what even my life coach could help me navigate. I knew I needed help, so I started going to regular therapy sessions to start processing and realigning my brain and nervous system after all the prolonged damage. Just like you need professionals to help heal a broken bone, you need trained mental health experts to recover from severe emotional and mental breaks.

In the previous chapter, we talked about the choices you have when you're living in trauma. Now it's time to examine the consequences and rewards of those choices. If you choose to stay, even if you start setting boundaries and getting support, there are still consequences to your physical, mental, and emotional well-being that will continue to some degree. You may gain coping skills, but the core issues remain. The trauma is still limiting your life.

However, if you make the difficult decision to leave an abusive situation, it opens the door for you to truly heal and overcome the effects of trauma so you can start to thrive. It's not an easy road and doesn't happen overnight—it takes consistent work and therapy and implementing new thought patterns and behaviors. But it allows you the opportunity to rediscover yourself, rebuild your health, and reclaim the life you deserve. There is so much to gain when you break free from trauma.

On the other hand, if you do nothing and remain paralyzed in a victim mentality, you lose twice. Not only do you have to keep living with all the current negative consequences, but you miss out on the potential of what your future could hold. Staying stuck steals your possibility. It's a double cost.

At this point, I'd encourage you to take an honest

assessment of how trauma has impacted you personally. How has it negatively affected your physical, mental, and emotional health? Where have you lost yourself and compromised your values? What parts of your personality have been overshadowed as you try to cope?

Really look at what it's costing you to keep enduring trauma and what you're forfeiting in the process—peace, joy, fulfillment, authenticity, health, purpose. Journal through it. Talk to a counselor or a trusted friend. Do the uncomfortable internal work to acknowledge the full scope of how it's holding you back and robbing you of your life. You have to face it to replace it.

Then ask yourself: Is this how I want to keep living? Am I willing to allow trauma to keep stealing from me or am I ready to take my life back? What will the consequences be for my future if I don't do anything? What opportunities and experiences will I miss out on? Who will I become if I don't break this cycle?

I know this deep dive into the repercussions of trauma is difficult. It's painful to see in black and white how much it has taken from you. But awareness is the first step to activating change. You can't address what you don't acknowledge. Give yourself grace and compassion as you get honest about where you are and how you're struggling. It's not your fault and it doesn't make you weak. Trauma is insidious and infiltrates even the strongest among us.

The good news is that healing and freedom are possible.

I'm living proof of that, even with how long I endured trauma and how far down it took me. No matter how much it has stolen, your future isn't shackled to your past. You can rise from the ashes and rebuild. You can get emotionally and mentally healthy. You can rediscover your strength and value. You can experience joy and peace again. But it starts with acknowledging the problem so you can take the first steps forward.

If this chapter resonated and you see how trauma has taken root in your mind and body, keep reading. In chapter five, we're going to talk about how to overcome the effects of trauma and rewire your brain and nervous system for health and wholeness. I'll share the strategies and practices that helped me break free from victimhood, rediscover my worth, and start living from a place of empowerment. Trauma doesn't get the final word. A new life awaits on the other side of healing.

Chapter 4 Homework

Go to God in prayer before you begin answering the following questions. Ask him to prepare you for this time and to share his wisdom and desires for your life.

1. Assess: Take a moment to consider your health. Which areas of your health have been neglected or are in poor condition due to your trauma?

2. Examine: What behaviors have you adopted from your toxic relationship or situation?
3. If you keep a journal what would you write today?
4. Identify: What resources or changes do you believe are necessary to achieve the life you dream of?
5. Analyze: How do you feel about your current situation? What steps do you want to take to change it?
6. Take Ownership: Reflect on your sense of control over your life. Do you feel like your trauma and toxicity have taken over and caused significant damage?
7. Explore: Have you changed any parts of your personality, your environment, or your aspirations to accommodate your traumatic situation? If so, how?
8. Inventory: How have changes in your circumstances negatively affected your physical, mental, and emotional health?
9. Reflect: Have you compromised your values because of your situation or surroundings? If so, how?

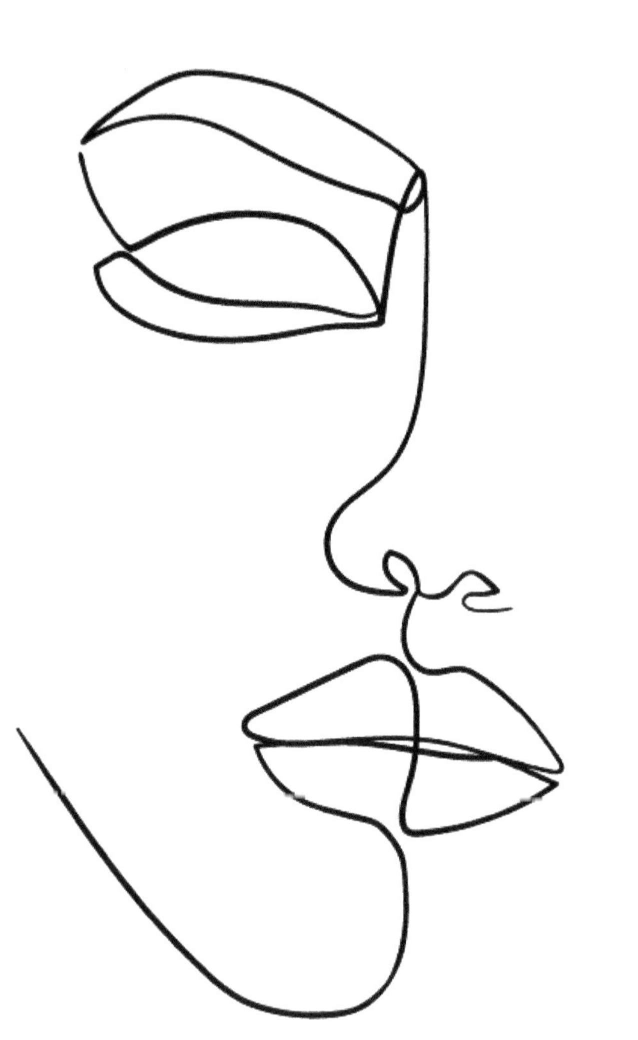

5

OVERCOMING TRAUMA

I sat on the porch of the cabin in Palo Duro Canyon, Texas, Bible open in my lap, taking slow deep breaths of the crisp morning air. My counselors at the intense marriage retreat had instructed each participant to spend time alone reflecting on the question: Who does God say you are? As I prayed and flipped through familiar scripture passages, a phrase seemed to jump off the page, speaking directly to my heart—"a chosen, priceless treasure."

Tears filled my eyes as I read the words again, letting their truth sink in. In God's eyes, I was his beloved child, an adopted daughter, cherished and valued beyond measure. Not because of anything I had done or achieved, but simply because He created me and chose me as his own. For the first time in years, a flicker of hope and purpose sparked deep within my soul.

I realized in that moment that if the God of the universe sees me as a priceless treasure, then that is what I need to base my entire self-worth and identity upon. Not the cruel words of my husband that had torn me down for decades. Not the trauma and betrayal that threatened to define me. But the steadfast love and delight of my Heavenly Father.

As I walked back to rejoin the group, I mulled over how viewing myself as God's priceless treasure should profoundly impact how I live my life. If I'm a priceless treasure, how should I be treating myself? What boundaries do I need to set? How should I expect others to speak to me and interact with me? Over the coming weeks and months, I determined to completely reorient my value system around this core, unshakable truth.

Healing and recovering from prolonged trauma is never a quick, easy journey. It's a winding path filled with ups and downs, victories and setbacks. Even after mustering the courage to leave my toxic marriage and start rebuilding my life, I still had an arduous road ahead learning to retrain my thoughts, behaviors, and emotions.

Overcoming trauma is not about breaking bad habits, but rather intentionally replacing them with healthy new ones. So, when negative self-talk would creep in, telling me I was unlovable and would never heal, I began the habit of reciting positive affirmations.

Every morning as I got ready for my day, I would look at myself in the mirror and declare these truths out loud: "Christel, you are a chosen, priceless treasure. You are beautiful, worthy, strong, and capable of incredible healing and purpose. Your past and your pain do not define you.

Each day you are becoming a braver, wiser, more joyful version of yourself."

Initially, these words felt hollow, and I struggled to believe them. But as I continued to faithfully repeat them day after day, I noticed my confidence and mood gradually improving. Just like building physical muscles, strengthening our mental and emotional muscles requires consistent effort and determination.

In addition to revamping my inner self-talk, I also had to retrain how I allowed others to treat me. For far too long I had tolerated unacceptable behavior from family, friends, and church members. Their constant criticisms, harsh judgments, and unhelpful advice reinforced my feelings of shame and hopelessness. I finally recognized that in order to heal and move forward, I needed to firmly establish new boundaries.

This meant having some difficult, direct conversations. Sometimes I had to limit or cut off contact completely with toxic people unwilling to respect my needs and boundaries. Other times, I had to repeatedly, calmly remind people when they made hurtful comments or violated the relational guardrails I had tried to establish. It felt incredibly uncomfortable and scary to speak up for myself after years of cowering. But it was also deeply empowering.

I soon realized that just as I was retraining my own behaviors and responses, I also needed to retrain the people in my life regarding what I would and would not tolerate. Very few made nasty remarks or attacked my character outright. But many still engaged in subtle digs, guilting or pressuring me to "get over it" and "move on" before I felt ready. Learning to identify those red flags and assert myself with both kindness and firmness was a major turning point.

Along with setting external boundaries, I had to dig deep to examine and reset my internal boundaries. What thoughts was I allowing my mind to dwell on? How much access was I giving my husband and the wounds of my past to my current emotional state? Just because a painful memory resurfaced, or I experienced a PTSD episode, didn't mean I had to be held captive by it for hours or days.

One particularly triggering incident during my healing process occurred while having coffee with a girlfriend. When our waiter politely leaned over to ask if he could clear our dirty dishes, I panicked. His unexpected close proximity and the sound of his voice caught me off guard, and I let out a scream. Logically I knew I was completely safe, but my body reacted as if I was back in the throes of trauma.

Through lots of counseling, I've learned techniques to help reverse those trigger spirals. Square breathing, grounding exercises, and visualizing myself in a peaceful, safe place help reset my equilibrium much faster. Progress hasn't been linear, and I still occasionally wake up in the middle of the night with anxiety attacks. But I no longer berate myself for it. I hold space for my body and brain to continue unlearning what kept me alive in survival mode for so long.

As I've released the heavy burdens of self-hatred, bitterness, and regret, I'm learning to embrace the "holy unraveling" as I call it. Deconstructing my old false beliefs, coping mechanisms, and ways of relating feels disorienting, and I often don't recognize myself. But I'm also experiencing a depth of peace, self-acceptance, and purpose I never dreamed possible.

Honestly, rewiring my brain to equate this lightness and ease with my new normal has been one of the biggest challenges. For decades, heaviness and hypervigilance were my constant companions, so when joy and spontaneous laughter bubble up from a deep well within me today, my knee-jerk response is "This feels so foreign. When will the other shoe drop?"

When I notice those old thoughts and emotions creeping in, I stop myself and acknowledge, "No, this is right and good. You are allowed to be happy and carefree. You don't have to earn it or wait for it to get yanked away at any moment. This is what true healing and freedom look like." Walking through the valley of the shadow of death with Jesus by my side has led me to spacious fields of wild, grateful wonder.

Looking back on the nine months I lived alone after leaving my husband, I can see what a sacred chrysalis that season was. Stripping everything away and getting reacquainted with my most basic needs, desires, feelings, and opinions felt awkward and scary but also thrilling. Who was I now? What did I enjoy? What did I want my new life to look and feel like? Pulling up so many old unhealthy roots and tenderly replanting beautiful new seeds of hope took immense patience and tenderness.

Just as a dormant bud can only blossom in the right conditions and timing, sustainable inner transformation refuses to be rushed. There is no magic formula or perfect timeframe for every person's healing journey. We each have our own unique layers and scars that require an abundance of perseverance and self-compassion to rehabilitate.

Remember to give yourself grace and release any illusion of "arriving" or crossing a finish line. Trauma recovery and becoming your truest, most whole self is a lifelong adventure and you will absolutely fall down, over and over again. But each time you get back up, dust yourself off, and realign toward your True North, you are making heroic strides.

You are not behind. You are not inadequate. You are right where you need to be and your messy, non-linear path is making you incomparably resilient and radiant from the inside out. When you feel overwhelmed by how far you still have to go, pause and look back at the view behind you. Haven't you come so much further than you ever dreamed you could? What an unspeakable privilege it is to be able to walk forward in freedom with your head held high!

Sometimes moving forward requires allowing yourself space to properly grieve and process the trauma you've endured. You may feel like you're taking two steps forward then one step back. And that's OK. Honor the reality that you've lost something precious—your sense of safety, identity, and trust. Squashing or rushing grief is never a good long-term strategy.

I love how Psalm 23 gives us language to pray during life's darkest valleys. "Yea, though I walk through the valley of the shadow of death, I will fear no evil; For You are with me; Your rod and Your staff, they comfort me. You prepare a table before me in the presence of my enemies." Our greatest enemies are often the sinister lies trauma has seared into our minds and our self-sabotaging habits. But over time, as we feast on God's promises, He redeems and transforms them for our good and His glory.

Take a minute to reflect. How is God inviting you to renew your thoughts and behaviors to align with your true worth and identity? What toxic cycles do you want to break in order to open space for vitality and beauty to bloom? What boundaries might you need to lovingly impose on yourself or others? Write down two or three small action steps you will take this week.

Dear reader, I know you've been through the unimaginable, and this uphill climb feels endless most days. But I'm here to cheer you on and remind you that you can do incredibly hard things. You were created on purpose, for a purpose, by a God who cherishes you as His beloved child. You are worth fighting for. You are worth believing in. Don't ever lose sight of the eternal value and glory your pain is producing. Keep going, one breath and baby step at a time. I'm rooting for you.

In the next chapter, we'll dive into the crucial question: "Who Do You Want to Be?" It's time to take back the pen of your story and become the hero you've been waiting for.

Chapter 5 Homework

Go to God in prayer before you begin answering the following questions. Ask him to prepare you for this time and to share his wisdom and desires for your life.

1. Pray: Spend time in God's word and reflect on your identity in His eyes. Who does God say you are?
2. Renew: How is God inviting you to renew your thoughts and behaviors to align with your true worth and identity?
3. Visualize: Envision yourself after setting boundaries or moving past the toxic situation you're in. What does this version of yourself look like?
4. Name: The likelihood we'll achieve our goals increases dramatically when we have an accountability partner. Who will you add to your support system to help keep you on track?
5. Identify: If you choose to stay in your situation and set new boundaries, who or what organization can you reach out to for guidance and help developing new habits?

6. Reframe: It often takes a shift in mindset to believe that you are who God says you are. What steps do you need to take to bring about this change in your thinking?
7. Examine: Spend time reflecting on your identity in the eyes of others and God, recognizing that His perspective is the truth. With this in mind, consider who you are now and who you aspire to be. You are not defined by your past trauma or your current circumstances.
8. Envision: Think about the person you want to become. What does this person look like? How does this person act? Describe her in detail.

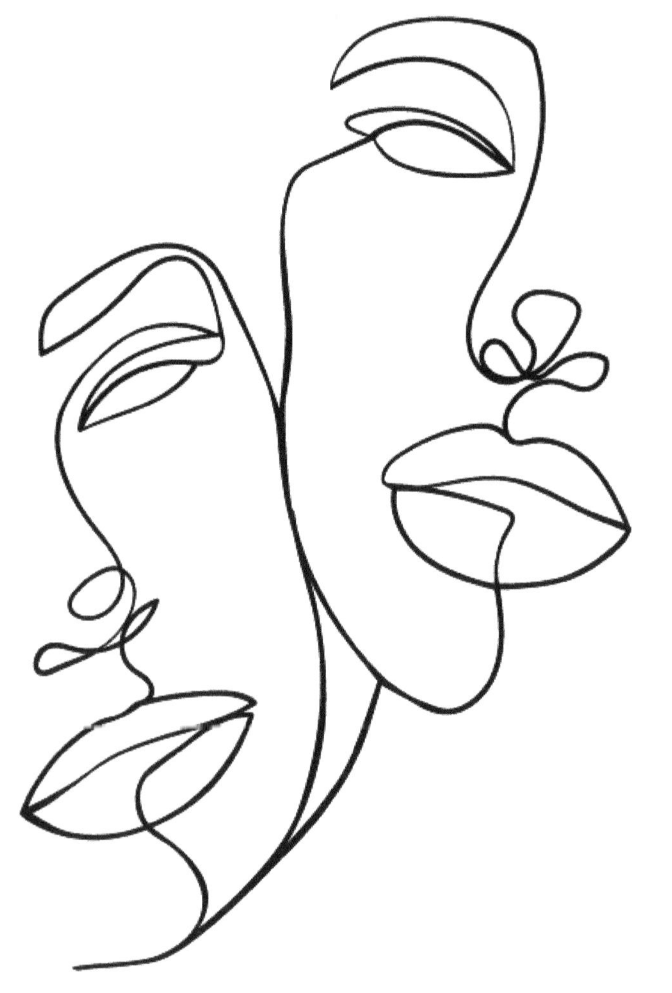

6

WHO DO YOU WANT TO BE?

As I sit here in my new home, surrounded by boxes still waiting to be unpacked, I can't help but reflect on the journey that brought me here. The journey of discovering who I truly am and who I want to be. It's a journey that began long before I ever realized it, a journey that was shaped by trauma and pain, but ultimately led me to a place of healing and self-discovery.

You see, when you've been through the kind of trauma that so many of us have experienced, it's easy to lose sight of who you are. It's easy to get caught up in the chaos and the pain, to let your identity be defined by the actions of others. But at some point, you have to make a choice. You have to decide who you're going to be after this, and you can't do it by yourself.

For me, that realization came slowly. It started when I moved away from my husband for four months to help my dad. During that time, I started to see glimpses of the person I could be. I liked who I was when I was away from the toxic environment of my marriage. But it wasn't until I started working with a counselor that things really began to change.

My counselor was the first person to validate my feelings. He told me that it was OK to feel the way I felt, to want what I wanted. That may seem like a small thing, but for someone who had been told for so long that my feelings didn't matter, it was a revelation. It was the turning point that made me realize I deserved better, that I could have the life I wanted.

But figuring out what that life looked like wasn't easy. It took work—a lot of work. I had to examine every area of my life and decide who I wanted to be in each one. I knew I wanted to be independent, successful, someone that people could look up to. I wanted to be someone that I could be proud of, someone that when I died and went home to God, He would look at me and say, "Well done, my good and faithful servant."

One of the hardest things for me was figuring out what I wanted in a relationship. After being in such a toxic marriage for so long, the idea of being in another relationship was terrifying. But I knew that eventually, I wanted to find someone to share my life with. So I started mapping out exactly what I was looking for in a partner.

I remember one time, a friend of mine was shocked when I turned down a date with a guy who had asked me out. She couldn't understand why I would say no. But the truth was, he didn't meet the new standards that I had set for myself. He noticed my friend first when he walked into the room, and that wasn't good enough for me. I knew my worth, and I wasn't going to settle for anything less than what I deserved.

You see, that's the thing that so many people struggle with—finding value in themselves. It's where our low self-esteem comes from. We've been told for so long that we're not good enough, that we don't deserve better. But the truth is, God tells us over and over again in the Bible that we are chosen. We are chosen by Him, but we're also chosen by the people in our lives—our employers, our spouses, our friends. When you start to see yourself as someone who is chosen, it changes everything.

But even with that knowledge, the journey to becoming who you want to be is not an easy one. There will be setbacks and obstacles along the way. There will be times when you feel like giving up, when you wonder if it's all worth it. But I promise you, it is.

You have to remember that you can't change anything that happened before. You have no control over what's going to happen in the future. All you have is right now, this moment. And in this moment, you have the power to choose who you want to be.

It's a choice that requires constant work and effort. You have to be willing to never stop learning, never stop growing. You have to prepare yourself physically, mentally, and emotionally for whatever comes your way. Because the truth is, life will always throw challenges at you. But if you've done the work, if you've prepared yourself, you'll be able to handle those challenges without being drained or overwhelmed.

For me, that work looks like a lot of different things. It looks like going to the gym even when I don't feel like it because I know that taking care of my physical health is important. It looks like reading books and listening to podcasts, constantly seeking out new knowledge and perspectives. It looks like surrounding myself with people who support and encourage me, who push me to be my best self.

But most importantly, it looks like constantly checking in with myself, asking myself if the choices I'm making align with the person I want to be. It's not always easy, and I don't always get it right. There are times when I slip up, when I make a choice that doesn't align with my values. But the important thing is that I don't let those slip-ups define me. I pick myself up, I learn from my mistakes, and I keep moving forward.

Because at the end of the day, that's what this journey is all about—moving forward. It's about letting go of the past, of the trauma and the pain that has held you back for so long. It's about embracing the present, and all the possibilities that it holds. And it's about looking to the future with hope and excitement, knowing that you have the power to create the life you want for yourself.

As I sit here in my new home, I'm filled with that hope and excitement. I know that there will be challenges ahead, that there will be times when I question myself and my choices. But I also know that I have the tools and the strength to face those challenges head-on. I know that I am not defined by my past, but by the choices I make in the present.

Looking ahead to the future, I am filled with a sense of possibility. I know that this is just the beginning of a new chapter in my life, a chapter that I get to write for myself. I am excited to see where this journey takes me and to continue becoming the person I want to be.

And so, to all of you out there who are struggling, who are feeling lost and alone, I want you to know that you are not alone. You are worthy of love and happiness, and you have the power to create the life you want for yourself. It won't be easy, and it will take work. But I promise you, it will be worth it.

So take a deep breath, and take that first step. Reach out to a professional who can help guide you on this journey. Surround yourself with people who support and encourage you. And most importantly, never stop believing in yourself. Because you are capable of amazing things, and the world needs the unique gifts and talents that only you can offer.

As we move forward into the next chapter, "A New Beginning," I want you to remember that every day is a chance to start anew. Every morning when you wake up, you have the opportunity to make choices that align with the person you want to be. And as you do that, day by day, choice by choice, you will begin to see yourself transform.

You will begin to become the person you were always meant to be.

Chapter 6 Homework

Go to God in prayer before you begin answering the following questions. Ask him to prepare you for this time and to share his wisdom and desires for your life.

1. Validation: Have you ever just wanted to be validated in your feelings? What areas of life do you need to feel validated in?
2. Self-Reflection: Ask yourself the next few questions to help you look into who you are and who you want to be.
3. Interests: What are your interests? (Not interests you have liked to please others, but truly yours)
4. Vision: What do you want your new life to look like?
5. Changes: What changes do you need to make to achieve your new life desires?
6. Time Frame: What time frame do you want to accomplish these changes?
7. Accountability: How, What, or Who will you use to help you be accountable to your goals and desires for change?
8. Progress Tracking: Create a positive way to track your progress and develop a way to give simple awards to yourself along the way.

9. Values and Boundaries: What values, standards, or boundaries will you set for yourself?
10. Self-Worth: What value do you see in yourself? Who does God say you are? What value does God see in you?
11. Self-Checks: How can you do self-checks to make sure you are always moving forward and healing?

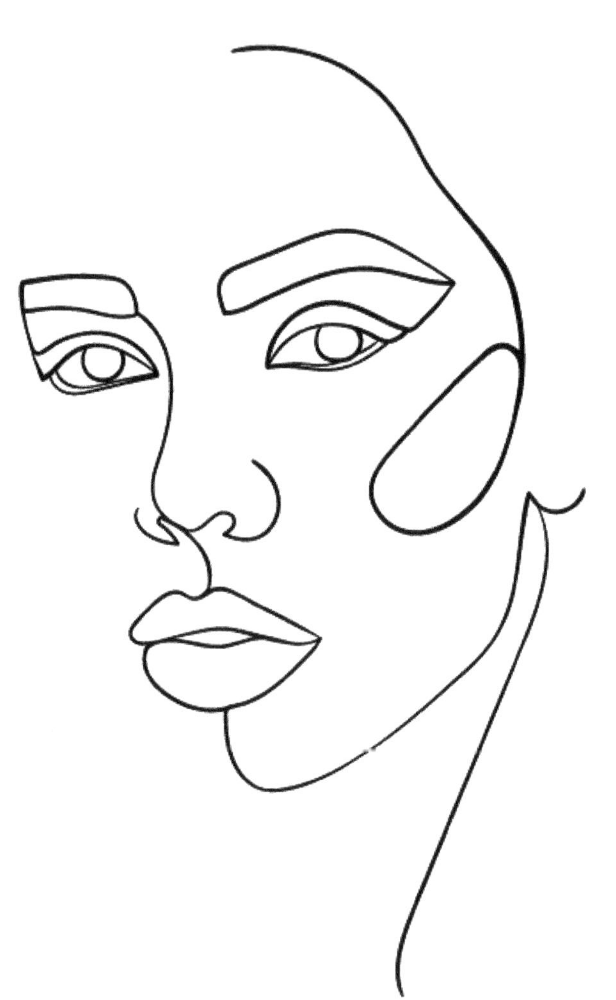

7

A NEW BEGINNING

Whether we choose to stay in our current situation or get out, a new beginning awaits us all. The person I was before the trauma no longer exists—physically, mentally, and emotionally, I have been transformed. It's up to each of us to decide who we want to become and carry that vision with us as we set new boundaries and live from a place of dignity and self-respect.

I remember my Sunday school teacher, Granny Vickers, telling me to keep the little booklet with the date of my salvation written inside. "When Satan comes to tell you that's not who you are," she said, "you have that to go back and remember, yes, it is who I am. And this is the day it happened."

In the same way, as we forge our new identities, we need to keep a clear picture of who we want to be. When I weighed 250 pounds, I started envisioning myself with an hourglass figure. I carried that image with me, and now, 100 pounds lighter, I am living proof that our minds can shape our realities.

Creating a vision board can be a powerful tool in this process. Fill it with images and words that represent the person you want to become—your ideal physical appearance, your emotional state, your intellect. Memorize the fruits of the Spirit—love, joy, peace, patience, kindness, goodness, and self-control—and work on embodying these qualities each day.

As I've walked this path, King David's story has been a constant source of inspiration. He wasn't perfect, but he's still known as a man after God's own heart. Like David, my road to change has been paved with both successes and failures, but each failure has been an opportunity to learn and grow.

What set David apart was that his heart was always in the right place. Despite his many failings—adultery, murder, a dysfunctional family— he never let these define him. Instead, he defined himself as a chosen child of God. This is a powerful lesson for all of us: No matter what we've been through, our past doesn't have to dictate our future.

So where do we start? The first step is to take an honest look at our lives and identify what brings us joy and what doesn't. Keep the things that make you happy, bless you, and bring you closer to the fruits of the Spirit. For the things that don't, ask yourself: Can I change them, or do I need to let them go?

This might mean changing jobs, moving to a new place, or ending toxic relationships. With each decision, ask yourself: Will this get me closer to my goal, or will it hold me back? It's not always easy, but choosing yourself is always worth it.

When I began this journey, I was afraid to be myself. But as I've gained confidence and learned to make different choices, I've found a freedom I never knew existed. I now expect the people around me to support and value me the way I value myself.

This shift in mindset didn't happen overnight. It took me years to get to where I am today, and there were plenty of times I felt discouraged and wanted to withdraw. But I kept coming back to the truth that I am a priceless treasure, worthy of love, respect, and happiness.

If I am a priceless treasure to myself, then it's my responsibility to protect the essence of who I am. This means prioritizing self-care, exercising, reading, furthering my education, and believing in myself. It means refusing to minimize my accomplishments or hide my intelligence to avoid intimidating others.

It means setting clear boundaries and not tolerating disrespect, secrecy, manipulation, or abuse from anyone—partners, family members, or friends. I expect to be treated as an equal in my relationships, and I surround myself with people who uplift and celebrate me sincerely.

I've learned to recognize one-sided relationships quickly and release them, choosing my emotional safety over familiarity or material security. While I understand that disagreements are a normal part of any relationship, I will not accept cruelty or contempt from those who claim to love me.

This has meant letting go of toxic friends and family members, which has been incredibly painful. But I know that in order to protect myself and teach my children about healthy boundaries, I must lead by example. I've had to release the guilt I feel over others' reactions to me putting myself first.

Never again will I accept violence as normal in a relationship, justify bad behavior, or make excuses for those who harm me. My time and energy are precious, and I refuse to waste them on people or situations that don't serve me.

I've learned to advocate for my needs and wants unapologetically and to walk away from any situation that feels similar to past abuse. I allow my deal-breakers to actually be deal-breakers, no matter how difficult it may be.

As I've grown in self-worth, I've had to fight the urge to overcompensate out of insecurity. I no longer bankroll others' lives or consistently pay more than my fair share. Instead, I share my story bravely when appropriate, in the hopes of helping others who are experiencing similar struggles.

Embracing my strength and resilience hasn't been easy, but it's been so worth it. I've come to realize that my dream relationship won't require me to change who I am at my core. I am releasing the fear of never measuring up and learning to embrace being perfectly imperfect.

When we learn to love and value ourselves, the possibilities are truly endless. Every day is a new opportunity to start over and make different choices. As someone who finds decision-making easy, I know this isn't the case for everyone. But even when we fail, we can still win if we learn from the experience.

As you step into your new beginning, remember this: Once you find out who you are and learn to like that person, it's OK if others don't. For years, I pretended not to be smart because I was afraid of intimidating people. But hiding our light only dims our own path.

Embracing your authentic self might feel awkward at first. It takes time for our nervous systems to adjust to feeling happy and having fun after trauma. But keep reminding yourself that you are healing and that discomfort is a sign of growth.

Don't ignore the red flags as you move forward. Trust your instincts and prioritize your emotional safety. There's no right or wrong way to do this—if it works for you and aligns with your values, that's all that matters.

Coming out of trauma, it's normal to feel afraid. But don't let that fear keep you stuck. Get out there and go for it. Follow where you believe God is leading you, and step into the life you deserve.

Above all, remember that you are good enough. You are a priceless treasure, worthy of love, respect, and joy. You deserve all the good things life has to offer, just like everyone else.

As I reflect on my journey, I am reminded of the Japanese art of kintsugi, where broken pottery is repaired with gold. The belief is that by embracing flaws and imperfections, you can create an even stronger, more beautiful piece of art.

This is how I see my own healing journey and the journey of every trauma survivor. We have been shattered by the things we've endured, but in picking up the pieces and putting ourselves back together, we have the opportunity to create something even more extraordinary.

The gold in our fractures represents the wisdom, resilience, and self-love we have gained through our experiences. It represents our decision to choose ourselves, to set boundaries, to change our mindsets, and to redefine our futures.

Like a kintsugi bowl, we will never be the same as we were before the trauma. But that doesn't mean we are broken beyond repair. In fact, our scars make us even more unique, beautiful, and strong.

To my fellow survivors, I want you to know that healing is possible. You have the power within you to create the life you want, to love yourself fiercely, and to thrive in the face of adversity.

It won't be easy, and it won't happen overnight. But by taking small steps each day—setting boundaries, practicing self-care, surrounding yourself with supportive people, and believing in your own worth—you will get there.

When we're young, we often have a vision of our adult lives. We dream big, and then life happens. We face challenges, interruptions, and trauma. But it's never too late to go after that big dream because deep down, our inherent purpose—blessed on our life the moment we were created—is still there waiting for us.

So get out there and live life to the fullest. Follow where God wants you to go and don't live in fear. Live in the hope of possibilities that are in front of you. Never forget that you are a priceless treasure, worthy of love, respect, and happiness. Your past does not define you, and your future is yours to create. Embrace your scars, honor your journey, and step into your new beginning with courage and hope.

I took back the pen to write my own story. Now it's your turn.

Chapter 7 Homework

Go to God in prayer before you begin answering the following questions. Ask him to prepare you for this time and to share his wisdom and desires for your life.

1. Identify: In the previous chapter, you looked at who you want to be. What is the first step you will take to become this person? When will you take this step?

2. Assess: What changes do you need to make to become this new version of yourself? Examples may include weight, job, friends, diet, exercise, and routine.
3. Plan: Are the timeframes and goals you've set for yourself realistic? How do you plan to hold yourself accountable to these goals?
4. Name: List three people or events from your life that have had a positive impact or left a lasting impression on you.
5. Journal: Throughout this process, journal your triggers regarding your traumatic responses to everyday situations in life. Understanding your triggers will facilitate changing and replacing your reactions.
6. Prepare: Identify two people you anticipate will have difficulty accepting the changes you are making in yourself. How can you maintain your boundaries and positive behavioral changes while navigating relationship obstacles with them?
7. Protect: Are there any friends or family members you may need to sever ties with for the sake of your mental health and stability?
8. Evaluate: Schedule a time to reevaluate yourself in approximately three to six months. If you achieve your goals by then, how will you reward yourself?

www.ingramcontent.com/pod-product-compliance
Ingram Content Group UK Ltd.
Pitfield, Milton Keynes, MK11 3LW, UK
UKHW021839270726
14058UKWH00002B/236